The Ultimate Anti-Inflammatory Diet Cookbook

Reduce Inflammation in the Body With Delicious Recipes

By
Olga Jones

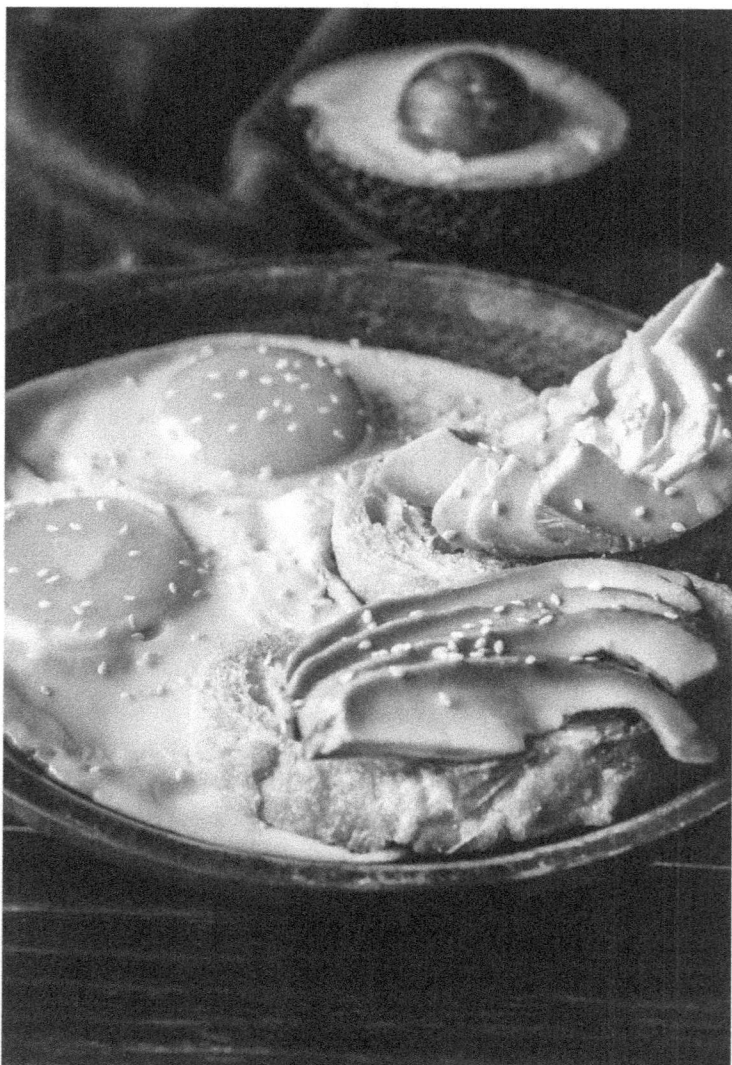

the publisher or the original author of this work can be in any fashion deemed liable for any hardship or damages that may befall them after undertaking information described herein.

Additionally, the information in the following pages is intended only for informational purposes and should thus be thought of as universal. As befitting its nature, it is presented without assurance regarding its prolonged validity or interim quality. Trademarks that are mentioned are done without written consent and can in no way be considered an endorsement from the trademark holder.

Table of Contents

INTRODUCTION

What is the Anti-Inflammatory Diet?

The anti-inflammatory diet is the best choice for your health if you have conditions that cause inflammation. Such conditions are asthma, chronic peptic ulcer, tuberculosis, rheumatoid arthritis, periodontitis, Crohn's disease, sinusitis, active hepatitis, etc. Along with medical treatment, proper nutrition is very important. An anti-inflammatory diet can help to reduce the pain from inflammation for a few notches. Such a diet isn't a panacea but a significant help in any treatment. Inflammation is a natural response of your body to infections, injuries, and illnesses. The classic symptoms of inflammation are redness, pain, heat, and swelling. Nevertheless, some diseases don't occur any symptoms. Such illnesses are diabetes, heart disease, cancer, etc. That's why we should care about our health permanently and an anti-inflammatory diet is one of the ways for it.

Inflammation is your immune system's response to injury or unwanted microbes in your body. It is a natural process and vital part of your body's healing process. When inflammation becomes systemic and chronic, however, it becomes a problem, and measures need to be taken. This type of inflammation serves no purpose, and can cause a lot of harm to the body.

This book has a LOT of recipes, and not every recipe might work for you. For example, if you're allergic to dairy or gluten, the recipes containing those ingredients will cause more harm than good. However, substitutions are possible for all of these, so you will be fine following this book as long as you keep an eye on the ingredients and use a bit of creativity where you have to! Once you understand the fundamentals of the diet, you will be fully equipped to create your own recipes from scratch!This is the most important information that you should know before starting a diet. Any diet is not a magic remedy for all diseases; it is a support for the body during a difficult time of treatment. Start your new healthy life from one small step and you will see the huge results within half a year. You can be sure that your body will be thankful to you by giving you a fresh look and energy for new achievements.

BREAKFAST

Quinoa Bread

Yield: 12 servings
Preparation Time: 10 minutes
Cooking Time: 1½ hours

Ingredients:
- 1¾ cups uncooked quinoa, soaked for overnight and rinsed
- ¼ cup chia seeds, soaked in ½ cup of water for overnight
- ½ teaspoon bicarbonate soda
- Salt, to taste
- ¼ cup extra virgin olive oil
- ½ cup water
- 1 tablespoon fresh lemon juice

Directions:
1. Preheat the oven to 320 degrees F.
2. Line a loaf pan using a parchment paper.In a mixer, add all ingredients and pulse approximately 3 minutes.
3. Place the amalgamation into the prepared loaf pan evenly.
4. Bake for approximately 1½ hours.
5. Remove from your oven and aside for around 30 minutes before removing from the loaf pan.

Carrot Bread

Yield: 8 serving
Preparation Time: 10 min
Cooking Time: 60 minutes

Ingredients:
- 2 cups almond meal
- 1 teaspoon organic baking powder
- 1 tablespoon cumin seeds
- Salt, to taste
- 3 organic eggs
- 2 tablespoons macadamia nut oil
- 1 tablespoon using apple cider vinegar
- 3 cups carrot, peeled and grated
- ½-inch little bit of fresh ginger, peeled and grated
- ¼ cup sultanas

Directions:

1. Preheat the oven to 350 degrees F.
2. Line a loaf pan with parchment paper.
3. In a sizable bowl, mix together almond meal, baking powder, cumin seeds and salt.
4. In another bowl, add eggs, nut oil and vinegar and beat till well combined.
5. Add egg mixture into flour mixture and mix till well combined.
6. Fold in remaining ingredients.

7. Place the mix into prepared loaf pan evenly.

8. Bake for around 1 hour.

Blueberry Muffins

Yield: 10 servings
Preparation Time: 10 minutes
Cooking Time: 22-25 minutes

Ingredients:

- 2½ cups almond flour
- 1 tablespoon coconut flour
- ½ tsp baking soda
- 3 tablespoons ground cinnamon, divided
- Salt, to taste
- 2 organic eggs
- ¼ cup coconut milk
- ¼ cup coconut oil
- ¼ cup maple syrup
- 1 tablespoon organic vanilla flavor
- 1 cup fresh blueberries

Directions:

1. Preheat the oven to 350 degrees F.
2. Grease 10 cups of a large muffin tin.
3. In a big bowl, mix together flours, baking soda, 2 tablespoons of cinnamon and salt.
4. In another bowl, add eggs, milk, oil, maple syrup and vanilla and beat till well combined.
5. Add egg mixture into flour mixture and mix till well combined.
6. Fold in blueberries.

7. Place a combination into prepared muffin cups evenly.

8. Sprinkle with cinnamon evenly.

9. Bake for approximately 22-25 minutes or till a toothpick inserted within the center is released clean.

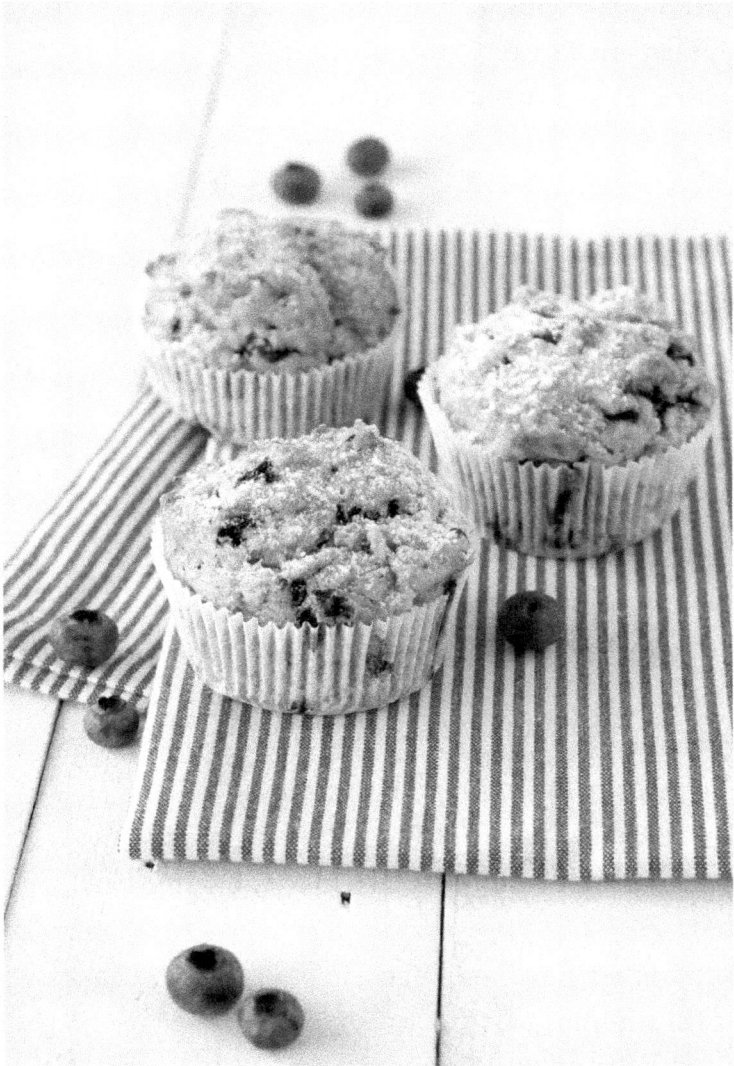

Savory Bread

Yield: 8-10 servings

Preparation Time: 10 minutes

Cooking Time: twenty or so minutes

Ingredients:
- ½ cup plus 1tablespoon almond flour
- 1 tsp. baking soda
- 1 teaspoon ground turmeric
- Salt, to taste
- 2 large organic eggs
- 2 organic egg whites
- 1 cup raw cashew butter
- 1 tablespoon water
- 1 tablespoon apple cider vinegar

Directions:

1. Preheat the oven to 350 degrees F.

2. Grease a loaf pan.

3. In a big pan, mix together flour, baking soda, turmeric and salt.

4. In another bowl, add eggs, egg whites and cashew butter and beat till smooth.

5. Gradually, add water and beat till well combined.

6. Add flour mixture and mix till well combined.

7. Stir in apple cider vinegar treatment.

8. Place the combination into prepared loaf pan evenly.

9. Bake for around twenty minutes or till a toothpick inserted within the center is released clean.

Crepes with Coconut Cream & Strawberry Sauce One

Preparation Time: quarter-hour Cooking Time: 8 minutes

Ingredients:

For Sauce:
- 12-ounces frozen strawberries, thawed and liquid reserved
- 1½ teaspoons tapioca starch
- 1 tablespoon honey For Coconut cream:
- 1 (13½- ounce) can chilled coconut milk
- 1 teaspoon organic vanilla flavoring
- 1 tablespoon organic honey

For Crepes:
- 2 tablespoons tapioca starch
- 2 tablespoons coconut flour •
- ¼ cup almond milk
- 2 organic eggs
- Pinch of salt
- Avocado oil, as required

Directions:

1. For sauce inside a bowl, mix together some reserved strawberry liquid and tapioca starch.
2. Add remaining ingredients and mix well.
3. Transfer a combination inside a pan on medium-high heat.
4. Bring to a boil, stirring continuously.

5. Cook for about 2-3 minutes or till sauce becomes thick.

6. Remove from heat and aside, covered till serving.

For coconut cream, carefully, scoop your cream from your surface of can of coconut milk.

1. In a mixer, add coconut cream, vanilla flavoring and honey and pulse for around 6-8 minutes or till fluffy.

1. For crepes in a blender, add all ingredients and pulse till well combined and smooth.

2. Lightly, grease a substantial nonstick skillet with avocado oil as well as heat on medium-low heat.

3. Add a modest amount of mixture and tilt the pan to spread it evenly inside the skillet.

4. Cook approximately 1-2 minutes.

5. Carefully, change the side and cook for approximately 1-1½ minutes more.

6. Repeat with the remaining mixture.

7. Divide the coconut cream onto each crepe evenly and fold into quarter.

8. Place strawberry sauce ahead and serve.

Honey Pancakes Satisfying

Yield: 2 servings
Preparation Time: 10 minutes
Cooking Time: 5 minutes

Ingredients:
- ½ cup almond flour
- 2 tablespoons coconut flour
- 1 tablespoon ground flaxseeds
- ¼ tsp baking soda
- ½ tablespoon ground ginger
- ½ tablespoon ground nutmeg
- ½ tablespoon ground cinnamon
- ½ teaspoon ground cloves
- Pinch of salt
- 2 tablespoons organic honey
- ¾ cup organic egg whites
- ½ teaspoon organic vanilla extract
- Coconut oil, as required

Directions:

1. In a big bowl, mix together flours, flax seeds, baking soda, spices and salt.

2. In another bowl, add honey, egg whites and vanilla and beat till well combined.

3. Add egg mixture into flour mixture and mix till well combined.

4. Lightly, grease a big nonstick skillet with oil and heat on medium-low heat.

5. Add about ¼ cup of mixture and tilt the pan to spread it evenly inside skillet.

6. Cook for about 3-4 minutes.

7. Carefully, customize the side and cook approximately 1 minute more.

8. Repeat with the remaining mixture.

9. Serve along with your desired topping.

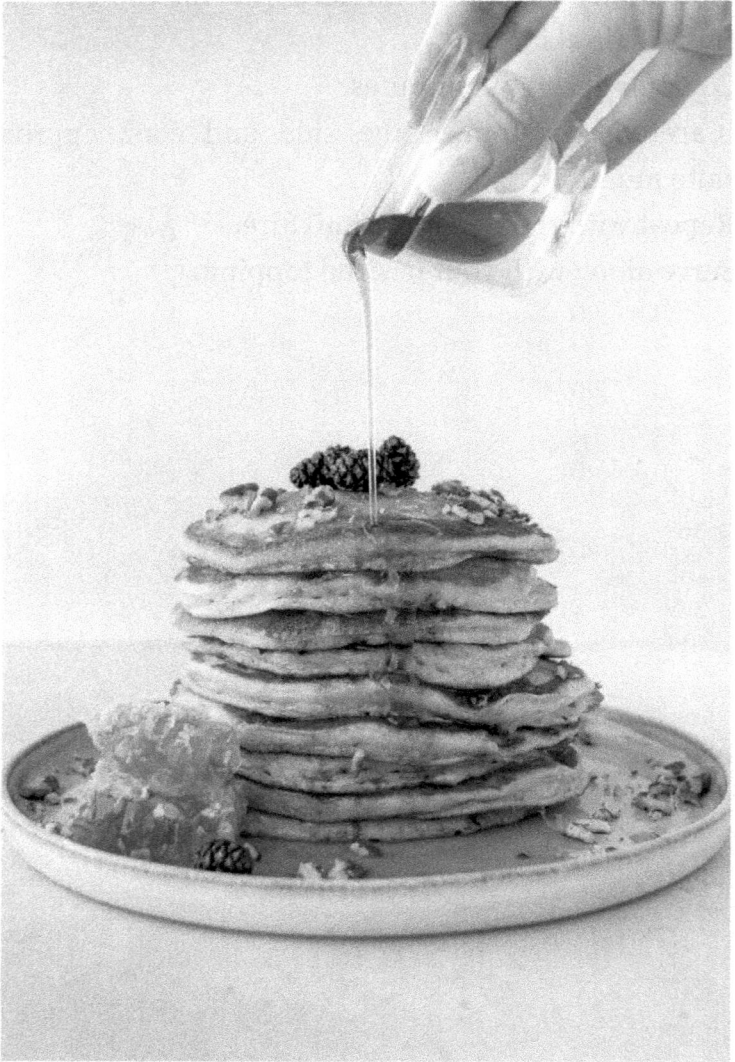

Zucchini Pancakes

Yield: 8 servings
Preparation Time: 15 minutes
Cooking Time: 6-10 min

Ingredients:
- 1 cup chickpea flour
- 1½ cups water, divided
- ¼ teaspoon cumin seeds
- ¼ tsp cayenne
- ¼ teaspoon ground turmeric
- Salt, to taste
- ½ cup zucchini, shredded
- ½ cup red onion, chopped finely
- 1 green chile, seeded and chopped finely
- ¼ cup fresh cilantro, chopped

Directions:
1. In a large bowl, add flour and ¾ cup with the water and beat till smooth.
2. Add remaining water and beat till a thin
3. Fold inside onion, ginger, Serrano pepper and cilantro.
4. Lightly, grease a substantial nonstick skillet with oil and heat on medium-low heat.
5. Add about ¼ cup of mixture and tilt the pan to spread it evenly in the skillet.
6. Cook for around 4-6 minutes.

7. Carefully, alter the side and cook for approximately 2-4 minutes.

8. Repeat while using remaining mixture.

9. Serve together with your desired topping.

Blueberry & Cashew Waffles

Yield: 5 servings
Preparation Time: quarter-hour
Cooking Time: 4-5 minutes

Ingredients:

- 1 cup raw cashews
- 3 tablespoons coconut flour
- 1 tsp baking soda
- Salt, to taste
- ½ cup unswee1oed almond milk
- 3 organic eggs
- ¼ cup coconut oil, melted
- 3 tablespoons organic honey
- ½ teaspoon organic vanilla flavor
- 1 cup fresh blueberries

Directions:

1. Preheat the waffle iron after which grease it.

2. In a mixer, add cashews and pulse till a flour like consistency forms.

3. Transfer the cashew flour in a big bowl.

4. Add almond flour, baking soda and salt and mix well.

5. In another bowl, add remaining ingredients and beat till well combined.

6. Add egg mixture into flour mixture and mix till well combined.

7. Fold in blueberries.

8. In preheated waffle iron, add required amount of mixture.

9. Cook for around 4-5 minutes.

10. Repeat with the remaining mixture.

Arugula & mushroom Frittata

Yield: 4-6 servings
Preparation Time: quarter-hour
Cooking Time: 23 minutes

Ingredients:
- ½ cup coconut milk
- 12 large organic eggs
- Salt, to taste
- 2 tablespoons coconut oil, divided
- 1 small red onion, chopped finely
- 1 cup fresh mushrooms, sliced
- 1 cup fresh arugula, chopped

Directions:
1. Preheat the oven to 375 degrees F.
2. In a bowl, add coconut milk, eggs and salt and beat well. Keep aside.
3. In an ovenproof skillet, heat 1½ tablespoons of oil on medium-high heat.
4. Add onion and sauté for approximately 3 minutes.
5. Add mushrooms and cook for around 6-8 minutes.
6. Add arugula and cook for approximately 2-3 minutes.
7. Transfer the vegetable mixture in a bowl.
8. In exactly the same pan, heat remaining oil on medium-low heat.
9. Add egg mixture and tilt the pan to spread the amalgamation evenly.
10. Cook for approximately 5 minutes.

11. Spread the vegetable mixture over cooked egg mixture evenly.

12. Immediately, transfer the skillet into oven.

13. Bake for about 5 minutes.

14. Remove from oven and carefully invert the frittata onto a plate.

15. Carefully, place within the skillet, cooked side up.

16. Bake for approximately 3-4 minutes more.

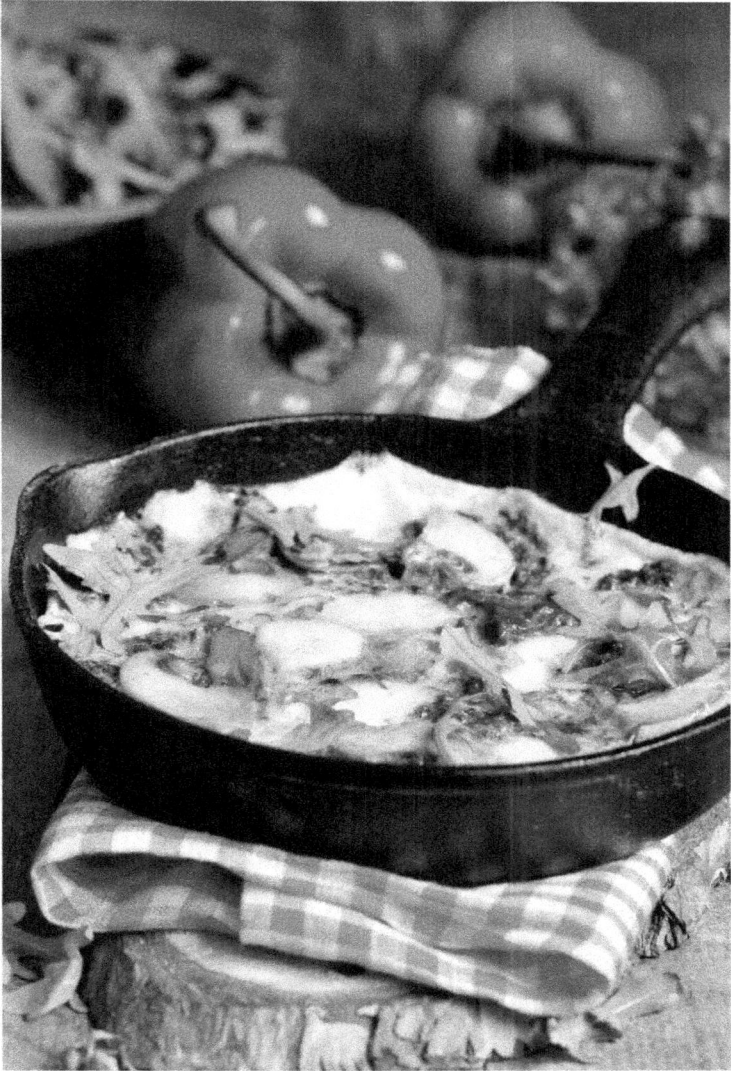

Baked Eggs with Spinach

Yield: 2 servings
Preparation Time: 15 minutes
Cooking Time: 22 minutes

Ingredients:
- 6 cups fresh baby spinach
- 2-3 tablespoons water
- 4 organic eggs
- Salt and freshly ground black pepper, to taste
- 2-3 tablespoons feta cheese, crumbled

Directions:
1. Preheat the oven to 400 degrees F.
2. Lightly, grease 2 small baking dishes.
3. In a substantial frying pan, add spinach and water on medium heat
4. Cook for approximately 3-4 minutes.
5. Remove from heat and drain the excess water completely.
6. Divide the spinach into prepared baking dishes evenly.
7. Carefully, crack 2 eggs in each baking dish over spinach.
8. Sprinkle with salt and black pepper and top with feta cheese evenly.
9. Arrange the baking dishes onto a big cookie sheet.
10. Bake for around 15-18 minutes.

LUNCH

Shrimp & Mango Salsa Lettuce Wraps

Yield: 6 servings
Preparation Time: 20 min
Cooking Time: 3 minutes

Ingredients:
For Salsa:
- 1 mango, peeled, pitted and chopped
- ¼ cup red onion, chopped finely
- ½ cup red bell pepper, seeded and chopped finely
- ¼ cup fresh cilantro, chopped
- 1 jalapeño pepper, seeded and chopped finely
- 2 tablespoons fresh lime juice •
- Salt and freshly ground black pepper, to taste

For Shrimp Wraps:
- 1 teaspoon organic olive oil
- 2 pounds large shrimp, peeled, deveined and chopped
- ½ teaspoon ground cumin
- 1 tablespoon red chili powder
- Salt and freshly ground black pepper, to taste
- 2 heads butter lettuce, leaves separated

Directions:

1. For salsa in a large bowl, mix together all ingredients. Keep aside.

2. In a big skillet, heat oil on medium heat.

3. Add shrimp and seasoning and cook for approximately 2-3 minutes.

4. Remove from heat and cool slightly.

5. Divide shrimp mixture over lettuce leaves evenly.

6. Top with mango salsa evenly and serve.

Bacon Wrapped Asparagus

Yield: 6 servings

Preparation Time: 10 min

Cooking Time: 25-a half-hour

Ingredients:

- 10 bacon slices, cut in half
- 1 pound fresh asparagus, trimmed
- 1 tablespoon extra virgin olive oil
- 1 tablespoon balsamic vinegar
- Freshly ground black pepper, to taste
- 1 lemon, sliced

Directions:

1. Preheat the oven to 400 degrees F. Line a substantial baking dish with foil paper.

2. Wrap one bacon slice around each asparagus piece.

3. Arrange asparagus in prepared baking dish.

4. Drizzle with oil and vinegar and sprinkle with black pepper.

5. Bake for approximately fifteen minutes. Change the inside and bake for 10-fifteen minutes more.

6. Serve immediately with lemon slices.

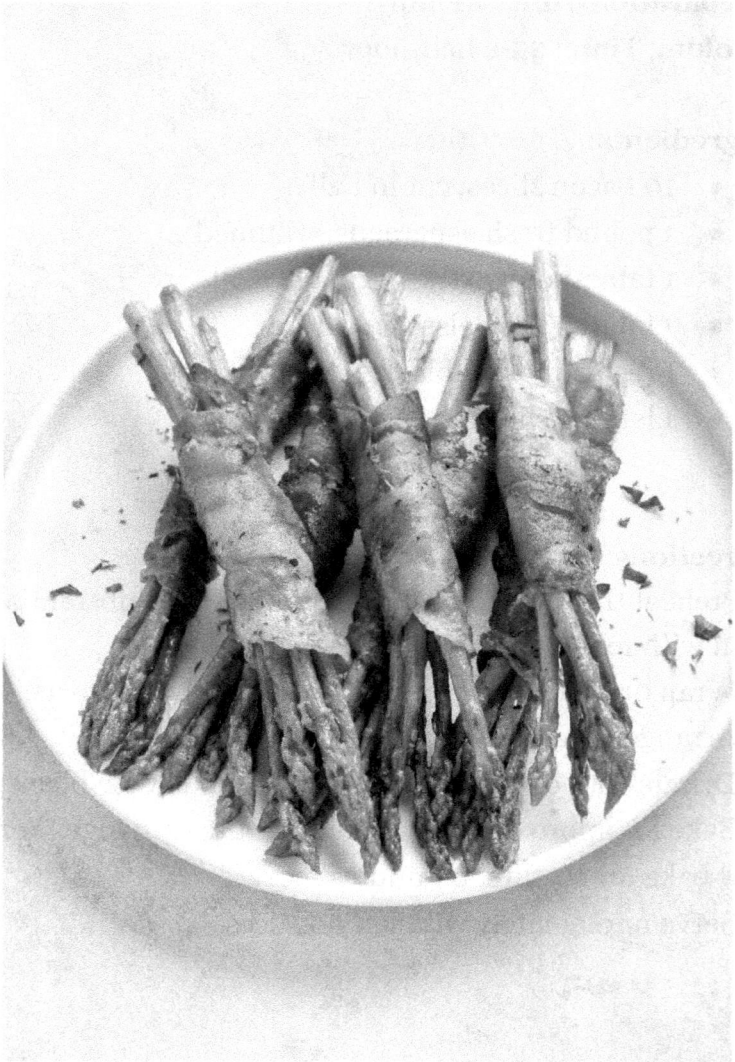

Zucchini Pasta With Shrimp

Yield: 4-6 servings

Preparation Time: 15 minutes

Cooking Time: 21 minutes

Ingredients:
- 2 tablespoons ghee or coconut oil
- 1 tablespoon extra virgin olive oil
- 3 garlic cloves, minced
- 1 pound shrimp, peeled and deveined
- 4 large zucchinis, spiralized with blade C
- Salt and freshly ground black pepper, to taste
- 4-6 fresh basil, eaves, chopped

Directions:

1. In a big skillet, heat ghee and essential olive oil on medium heat.

2. Add garlic and sauté approximately 1 minute.

3. Add shrimp and cook for approximately 2- 3 minutes.

4. Add zucchini, tossing occasionally and cook approximately 2-3 minutes.

5. Stir in salt and black pepper and take off from heat.

6. Serve while using garnishing of basil leaves.

Sweet Potato Buns Sandwich

Yield: 1 serving

Preparation Time: fifteen minutes

Cooking Time: 19 minutes

Ingredients:

For Sweet Potato Buns:

- 1½ tablespoons extra virgin olive oil, divided
- 1 large sweet potato, peeled and spiralized with blade C
- 2 teaspoons garlic powder
- Salt and freshly ground black pepper, to taste
- 1 large organic egg
- 1 organic egg white

For Sandwich:

- 1½-ounce salmon piece
- Salt and freshly ground black pepper, to taste
- 1 teaspoon fresh lime juice
- 1 tomato slice
- 1 onion slice
- ½ of an avocado, peeled, pitted and chopped
- 2 teaspoons fresh cilantro, chopped
- 1 large bit of fresh kale
- 1 bacon piece

Directions:

1. For buns in a sizable skillet, heat ½ tablespoon of oil on medium heat. 2

2. Add sweet potato and sprinkle with garlic powder, salt and black pepper.

3. Cook for 5-7 minutes. Transfer the sweet potato mixture into a bowl.

4. Add egg and egg white and mix well. Now, transfer a combination into 2 (6-ounce) ramekins, midway full.

5. Cover the ramekins with wax paper. Now, place over noodles and press firmly down. 6.Refrigerate for about 15-20 minutes.

7. Preheat the grill to medium heat. Grease the grill grate.

8. Meanwhile in a very bowl, add salmon, salt, black pepper and lime juice and toss to coat well.

9.In a substantial skillet, heat remaining oil on medium-low heat. Carefully, transfer the sweet 10.potato patties into skillet. Cook for 3-4 minutes. Change the medial side and cook for two-3 minutes more.

11.Place salmon, onion and tomato slices over grill.

12.Grill tomato slice for 1 minute. Grill onion slice for approximately 2 minutes.

13.Grill the salmon for approximately 4-5 minutes or till desired doneness.

14.In a bowl, add avocado and cilantro and mash well.

15. In a plate, place one sweet potato bun. Place onion slice, salmon, tomato, bacon and kale over bun.

16. Spread avocado mash around the bottom side of another bun. Place the bun, avocado mash side downwards over kale.

17. Secure using a toothpick and serve.

Shrimp, Sausage & Veggie Skillet

Yield: 4 servings
Preparation Time: 15 minutes
Cooking Time: 13 minutes

Ingredients:

- 3 tablespoons organic olive oil, divided
- 1 pound shrimp, peeled and deveined
- 2 teaspoons old bay seasoning •
- ½ of medium yellow onion, chopped
- ¾ cup green peppers, seeded and chopped
- ¾ cup green peppers, seeded and chopped
- 1 zucchini, chopped
- 6-ounces cooked sausage, chopped
- 2 garlic cloves,minced
- ¼ cup chicken broth
- Pinch of red pepper flakes, crushed
- Salt and freshly ground black pepper, to taste

Directions:

1. In a sizable skillet, heat 1 tablespoon of oil on medium-high heat.
2. Add shrimp and cook for around 3-4 minutes. Transfer the shrimp into a bowl.
3. In the identical skillet, heat remaining oil on medium heat.
4. Add onion and sweet peppers and sauté for about 4-5 minutes.

5. Add zucchini and sausage and cook for approximately 2 minutes.

6. Add garlic and cooled shrimp and cook for approximately 1 minute.

7. Add broth and stir to combine well. Stir in red pepper flakes, salt and black pepper and cook for approximately 1 minute.

8. Serve hot.

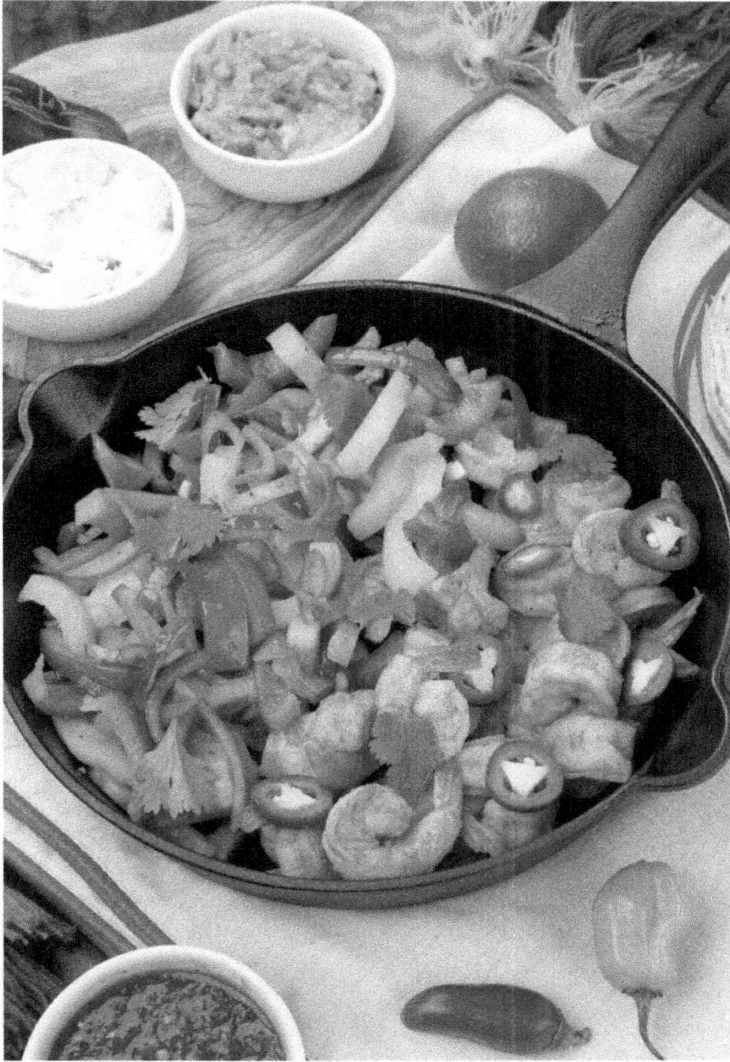

Sea Scallops With Spinach & Bacon

Yield: 4 servings

Preparation Time: quarter-hour

Cooking Time: 21 minutes

Ingredients:

- 3 bacon slices
- 1½ pound jumbo sea scallops
- Salt and freshly ground black pepper, to taste
- 1 cup onion, chopped • 6 garlic cloves, minced
- 12-ounces fresh baby spinach

Directions:

1. Heat a sizable nonstick skillet on medium-high heat.
2. Add bacon and cook for approximately 8-10 min.
3. Transfer the bacon into a bowl, reserving
4. 1 tablespoon of bacon Fat within the skillet.
5. Chop the bacon and keep aside.
6. Add scallops and sprinkle with salt and black pepper.
7. Immediately, boost the heat to high heat.
8. Cook for about 5 minutes, turning once after 2½ minutes. 9
9. Transfer the scallops into another bowl. Cover having a foil paper to ensure that they're warm.
10. In exactly the same skillet, add onion and garlic minimizing the temperature to medium-high.
11. Sauté onion and garlic for around 3 minutes.

12. Add spinach and cook for approximately 2-3 minutes. Season with salt and black pepper and remove from heat.

13. Divide the spinach among serving plates. Top with scallops and bacon evenly. Serve immediately.

Liver With Onion & Parsley One

Yield: 2-4 servings
Preparation Time: 10 minutes
Cooking Time: 26 minutes

Ingredients:
- 3 tablespoons coconut oil, divided
- 2 large onions, sliced
- Salt, to taste
- 1 pound grass-fed beef liver, cut into ½-inch thick slices
- Freshly ground black pepper, to taste
- ½ cup fresh parsley, chopped
- 2 tablespoons freshly squeezed lemon juice

Directions:
1. In a sizable skillet, heat 1 tablespoon of oil on high heat.
2. Add onion plus some salt and sauté for about 5 minutes.
3. Reduce the warmth to medium. Sauté the onion for 10-15 minutes.
4. Transfer the onion right into a plate.
5. In exactly the same skillet, heat another 1vtablespoon of oil on medium-high heat.

6. Add liver and sprinkle with salt and black pepper. Cook for approximately 1-1½ minutes or till browned.

7. Flip alongside it and cook for approximately 1-1½ minutes or till browned.

8. Transfer the liver right into a plate.

9. In the same skillet, heat remaining oil on medium heat.

10. Add cooked onion, parsley and lemon juice and stir well. Cook for about 2-3 minutes.

11. Place onion mixture over liver and serve immediately.

Egg & Avocado Wraps

Yield: 5 servings
Preparation Time: 20 minutes

Ingredients:
- 1 ripe avocado, peeled, pitted and chopped
- 1 tablespoon freshly squeezed lemon juice
- 1 tablespoon fresh parsley, chopped
- 2 tablespoons celery stalk, chopped
- 4 organic hard-boiled eggs, peeled and chopped finely
- Salt and freshly ground black pepper, to taste
- 4-5 endive bulbs
- 2 cooked bacon slices, chopped

Directions:
1. In a bowl, add avocado and freshly squeezed lemon juice and mash till smooth and creamy.
2. Add parsley, celery, eggs, salt and black pepper and stir to mix well.
3. Separate the endive leaves. Divide the avocado mixture over endive leaves evenly.
4. Top with bacon evenly and serve immediately.

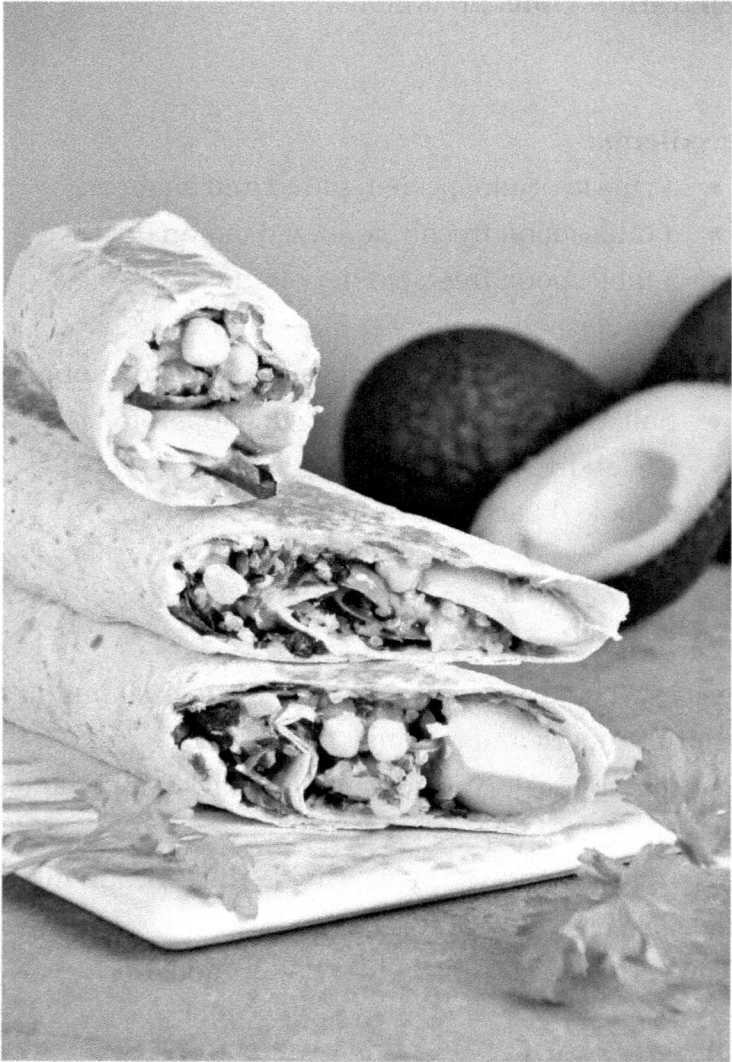

Prosciutto Wrapped Chicken

Yield: 8 servings

Preparation Time: 10 min

Cooking Time: 26 minutes

Ingredients:

- 3 tablespoons plus 1 teaspoon coconut oil, melted and divided
- 2 garlic cloves, minced
- 1 teaspoon fresh lemon zest, grated finely
- 1 tablespoon fresh lemon juice
- Salt, to taste
- 8 grass-fed skinless, boneless chicken thighs
- 8 sprigs fresh rosemary
- 8 prosciutto slices

Directions:

1. Preheat the oven to 400 degrees F. Arrange a big baking rack onto a big baking dish.

2. In a substantial bowl, add 3 tablespoon of coconut oil, garlic, lemon zest, fresh lemon juice and salt and mix till well combined.

3.Add chicken thighs and cot with mixture generously. Keep aside approximately 10 min.

4. Remove chicken thighs from mixture. Place 1 rosemary sprig within the center of each and every thigh and then then fold each thigh in half.

5. Wrap a prosciutto slice around each thighs tightly.

6. In a sizable skillet, heat remaining oil on medium high heat.

7. Add thighs and cook approximately 3 minutes per side.

8. Now, transfer thighs in prepared baking dish in the single layer.

9. Bake for approximately 18-twenty minutes.

Creamy Sweet Potato Pasta With Pancetta

Yield: 4 servings

Preparation Time: 15 minutes

Cooking Time: 21 minutes

Ingredients:

For Creamy Sauce:

- 4-5 cups cauliflower florets
- 1 small shallot, minced
- 1 large garlic herb, chopped
- Pinch of red pepper flakes, crushed
- 1 cup chicken broth
- 1 tablespoon nutritional yeast
- Sat, to taste • For Pancetta:
- 8 pancetta slices, cubed
- For Sweet Potato Pasta:
- 1 tablespoon extra-virgin olive oil
- 3 medium sweet potato, peeled and spiralized with blade C
- 3 cups leeks, chopped
- Salt and freshly ground black pepper, to taste
- 1 tablespoon fresh parsley, chopped

Directions:

1. In a pan of salted boiling water, add broccoli florets and cook for around 7-8 minutes. Drain well.

2. Meanwhile in heat a large nonstick skillet on medium heat.

3. Add pancetta slices and cook for approximately 5-7 minutes.

4. Transfer pancetta into a bowl.

5. In the identical skillet, add shallot, garlic and red pepper flakes and sauté for around 2 minutes.

6. Transfer the shallot mixture into a higher speed blender.

7. Add cauliflower and remaining sauce ingredients and pulse till smooth and creamy.

8. In the identical skillet, heat extra virgin olive oil on medium heat.

9. Add sweet potato and leeks and cook, tossing occasionally for approximately 8-10 min.

10. Stir in sauce and cook for about 1 minute.

11. Serve this creamy pasta with all the topping of pancetta and parsley.

Roasted Beet Pasta With Kale & Pesto

Yield: 3 servings
Preparation Time: quarter-hour
Cooking Time: 21 minutes

Ingredients:
For Pesto:

- 3 cups fresh basil leaves
- 1 large garlic oil
- ¼ cup organic olive oil
- ¼ cup pine nuts, chopped
- Salt and freshly ground black pepper, to taste
- For Beet Pasta:
- 2 medium beets, trimmed, peeled and spiralized with blade C
- Olive oil cooking spray, as required
- Salt and freshly ground black pepper, to taste For Kale:
- 2 cups fresh baby kale

Directions:

1. Preheat the oven to 425 degrees F. Lightly, grease a large baking sheet.
2. In a mixer, add all pesto ingredients and pulse till smooth. Keep aside.
3. Place beet pasta in prepared baking sheet.

4. Drizzle with cooking spray and sprinkle with salt and black pepper and gently, toss to coat well.

5. Roast for around 5-10 minutes or till desired doneness.

6. Transfer the pasta in a sizable bowl.

7. Add kale and pesto and gently, toss to coat well.

Veggies & Apple With Orange Sauce

Yield: 4 servings
Preparation Time: quarter-hour
Cooking Time: 16 minutes

Ingredients:
For Sauce:
- 1 (1-inch) fresh ginger, minced
- 2 garlic cloves, minced
- 1 tablespoon fresh orange zest, grated finely
- ½ cup fresh orange juice
- 2 tablespoons white wine vinegar
- 2 tablespoons coconut aminos
- 1 tablespoon red boat fish sauce

For Veggies & Apple:
- 1 tablespoon extra virgin olive oil
- 1 cup carrot, peeled and julienned
- 1 head broccoli, cut into florets
- 1 cup celery, chopped
- 1 cup onion, chopped
- 2 apples, cored and sliced

Directions:

1. In a sizable bowl, mix together all sauce ingredients. Keep aside.

2. In a big skillet, heat oil on medium-high heat.

3. Add carrot and broccoli and stir fry for about 4-5 minutes.

4. Add celery and onion and stir fry for approximately 4-5 minutes.

5. Pour sauce and stir to combine. Cook approximately 2-3 minutes.

6. Stir in apple slices and cook for about 2-3 minutes more.

7. Serve hot.

Cauliflower Rice With Prawns & Veggies

Yield: 4 servings
Preparation Time: 15 minutes
Cooking Time: 21 minutes

Ingredients:
- 2 tablespoons coconut oil, divided
- 14 prawns, peeled and deveined
- 2 organic eggs, bea10
- 1 brown onion, chopped
- 1 garlic cloves, minced
- 1 small fresh red chili, chopped
- ½ pound grass-fed ground chicken
- 1 cauliflower head, cut into florets, processed like rice consistency
- ¼ of red cabbage, chopped • ½ cup green peas, shelled
- 1 head small broccoli, cut into small florets

- 1 large carrot, peeled and chopped finely
- 1 small red bell pepper, seeded and chopped
- 2 bok choy, sliced thinly
- 3 tablespoons coconut aminos
- Salt and freshly ground black pepper, to taste

Directions:
1. In a substantial skillet, heat ½ tablespoon of oil on medium-high heat.
2. Add prawns and cook for approximately 3-4 minutes. Transfer in a large bowl.
3. In exactly the same skillet, heat ½ tablespoon of oil on medium heat.
4. Beat 10 eggs and with the back of a spoon, spread the eggs. Cook for around 2 minutes.
5. Remove eggs from skillet and cut into strips.
6. In the identical skillet, heat remaining oil on high heat. Add onion, garlic and red chili and sauté for about 4- 5 minutes.
8. 7. Add chicken and cook for about 4-5 minutes.
9. Add cauliflower rice and remaining veggies except bok choy and coconut aminos and cook for around 2-3 minutes.
10. Add bok choy, coconut aminos, cooked eggs, prawns, salt and black pepper and cook for 2 minutes more.

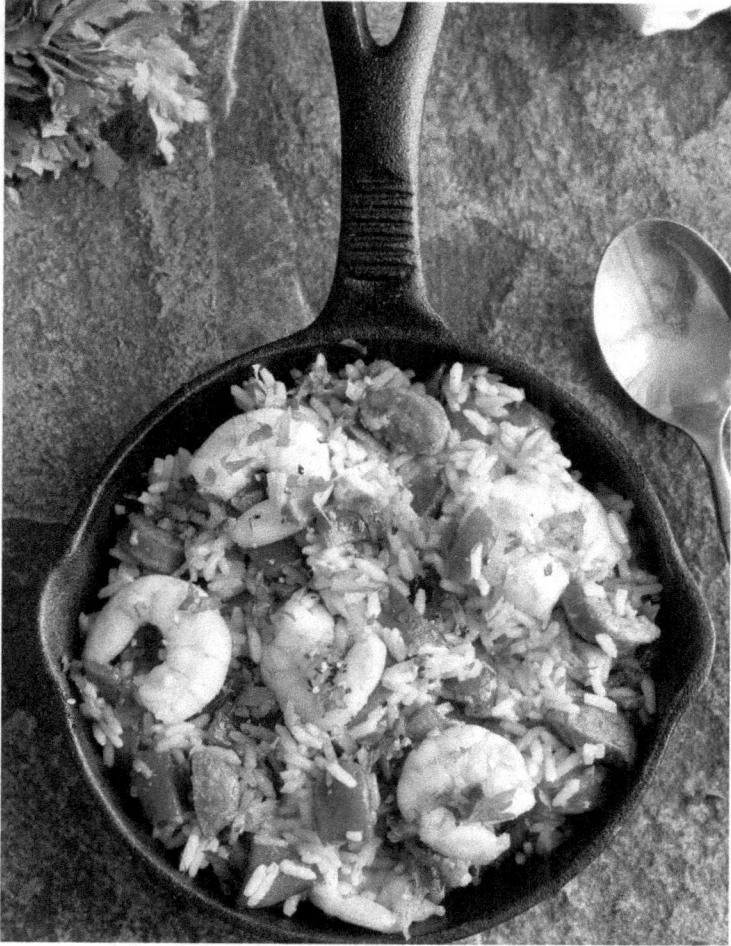

SMOOTHIES AND DRINKS

Almond Blueberry Smoothie

Time To Prepare: ten minutes

Time to Cook: 0 minutes

Yield: Servings 1

Ingredients:
- 1 banana
- 1 cup frozen blueberries
- 1 tbsp. almond butter 1
- /2 cup almond milk
- Water, as required

Directions:

1. Put in everything in a blender jug.

2. Cover the jug firmly.

3. Blend until the desired smoothness is achieved. Serve and enjoy!

Apple Cinnamon Water

Time To Prepare: five minutes
Time to Cook: five minutes
Yield: Servings 4

Ingredients:

- 1 whole apple, diced 5 cinnamon sticks Water to cover contents

Directions:

1. Put ingredients in the steamer basket.
2. Put in a pot. Put in water cover contents.
3. Secure the lid. Cook on HIGH pressure for five minutes.
4. When done, depressurize swiftly.
5. Remove steamer basket.
6. Discard cooked produce.
7. Let flavored water cool.
8. Chill completely before you serve

Beet and Cherry Smoothie

Time To Prepare: five minutes

Time to Cook: 0 minutes

Yield: Servings 4

Ingredients:

- ½ cup frozen cherries, pitted ½ teaspoon frozen banana
- 1 tablespoon almond butter 10-ounce almond milk, unsweetened 2 small beets, peeled and slice into four

Directions:

1. Put in all ingredients in a blender.
2. Blend until the desired smoothness is achieved.

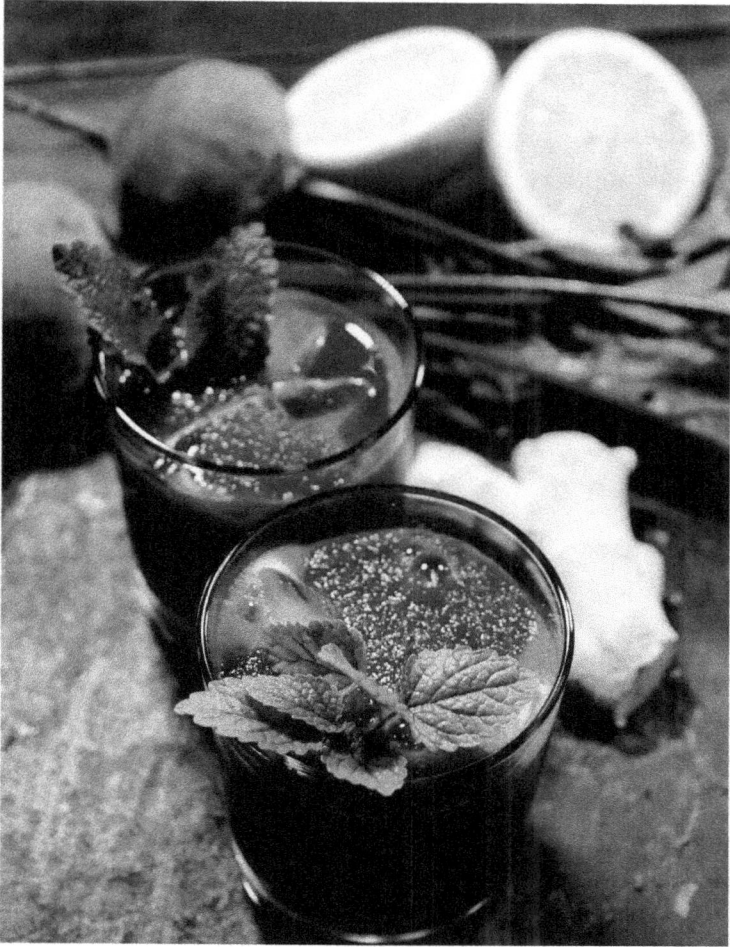

Berry Shrub

Time To Prepare:ten minutes

Time to Cook: twenty minutes

Yield: Servings 4

Ingredients:
- ½ a cup of chopped fresh oregano
- 1 cup of dried elderberries
- 2 cups of apple
- cider vinegar
- 2 cups of honey
- 2 cups of water

Directions:

1. Put in listed ingredients to the instant pot. Secure the lid.

2. Cook on HIGH pressure for twenty minutes.

3. When done, depressurize naturally.

4. Pour ingredients through a sieve into a jar. Let cool down. Chill.

Blackberry Italian Drink

Time To Prepare:five minutes
Time to Cook: fifteen minutes
Yield: Servings 4

Ingredients:
- 1 bottle sparkling water
- 1 cup blackberries
- 1 lemon, cut
- 2 tbsp. Honey

Directions:

1. Put in 1 cup (non-carbonated) water to the instant pot.

2. Put in blackberries to the instant pot. Secure the lid. Cook on HIGH pressure for ten minutes.

When done, depressurize naturally.

3. Mash the berries in the instant pot. Move to dish. Let cool.

4. As blackberries cook, in a separate small deep cooking pan with a heavy bottom.

5. Put in honey. Simmer for five minutes. Cool down.

6. To make the drink. Ladle 1 teaspoon honey. Pour in fruit mixture. Put in carbonated water. Stir.

Blueberry And Spinach Shake

Time To Prepare: five minutes

Time to Cook: 0 minutes

Yield: Servings 2

Ingredients:

- 1 cup of low-fat Greek yogurt (not necessary)
- 1 cup of organic blueberries (or washed if non-organic)
- 1/2 cup of spinach ice cubes to the desired concentration

Directions:

Put in ingredients together in a blender until the desired smoothness is achieved and then serve in a tall glass. Drizzle a few fresh berries on top if you prefer!

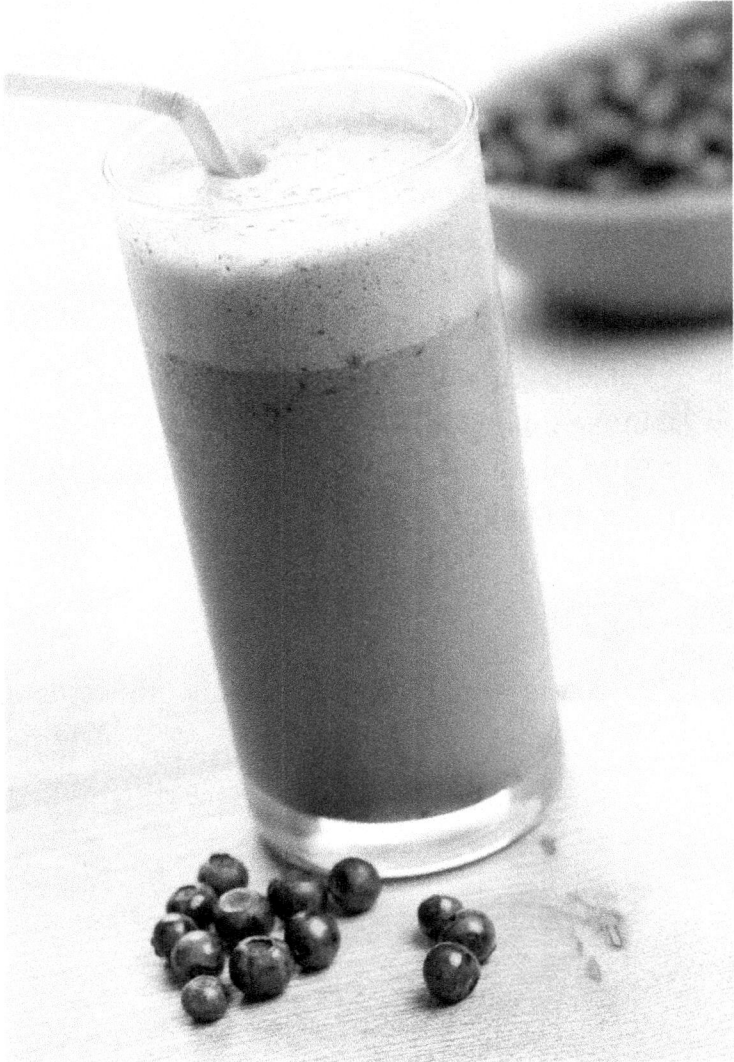

Blueberry Matcha Smoothie

Time To Prepare: five minutes

Time to Cook: 0 minutes

Yield: Servings 2

Ingredients:

- ¼ Teaspoon Ground Cinnamon
- ¼ Teaspoon Ground Ginger
- 1 Banana
- 1 Tablespoon Chia Seeds
- 1 Tablespoon Matcha Powder
- 2 Cups Almond Milk
- 2 Cups Blueberries, Frozen 2 Tablespoons Protein Powder, Optional A Pinch Sea Salt

Directions:

Blend all ingredients until the desired smoothness is achieved.

Blueberry Smoothie

Time To Prepare: ten minutes

Time to Cook: 0 minutes

Yield: Servings 1

Ingredients:
- 1 banana, peeled
- 1 tbsp. almond butter
- 1 tsp. maca powder
- 1/2 cup almond milk, unsweetened
- 1/2 cup blueberries
- 1/2 cup water
- 1/4 tsp. ground cinnamon
- 2 handfuls baby spinach

Directions:

In your blender, combine the spinach with the banana, blueberries, almond butter, cinnamon, maca powder, water, and milk. Pulse thoroughly, pour into a glass, before you serve. Enjoy!

Carrot and Orange Turmeric Drink

Time To Prepare: five minutes

Time to Cook: 0 minutes

Yield: Servings 2

Ingredients:

- 1 cup orange juice
- 1 tbsp. lemon juice
- 1/2 inch ginger slice
- 1/4 tsp. turmeric powder
- 2 carrots, peeled, chopped
- 2 tbsp. sugar

Directions:

In a blender, put in orange juice, sugar, turmeric powder, carrots, and lemon juice. Blend well. Serve!

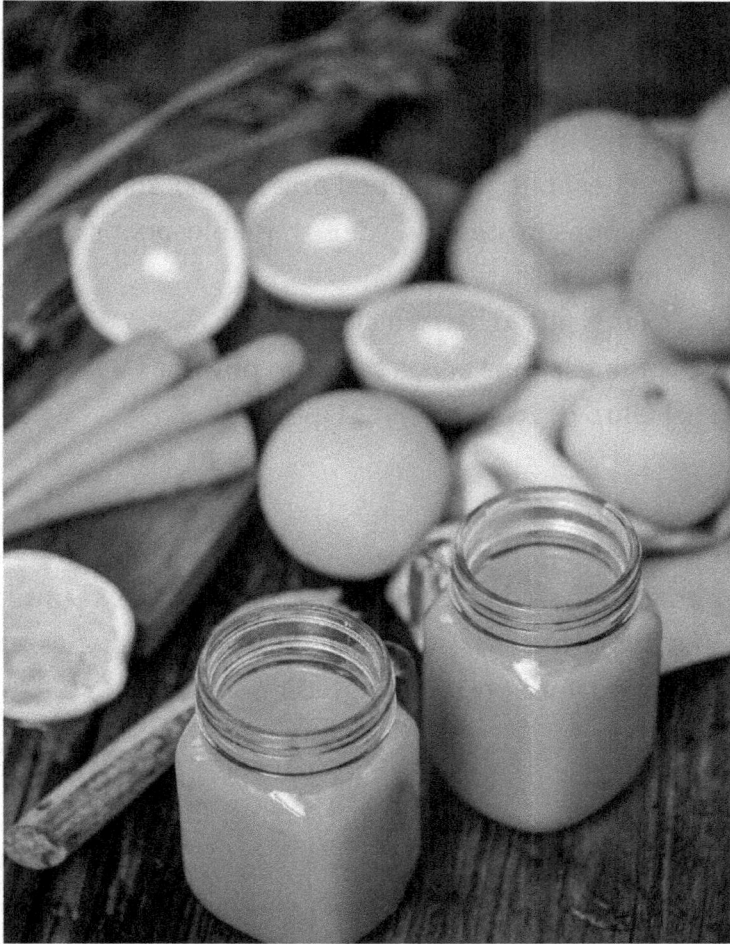

Chocolate Cherry Smoothie

Time To Prepare: five minutes

Time to Cook: 0 minutes

Yield: Servings 2

Ingredients:

- 2 cups almond milk, unsweetened
- 2 dates, pitted, chopped or 2 teaspoons pure maple syrup
- 2 scoops protein powder or 4 tablespoons almond butter (not necessary)
- 4 cups pitted, frozen cherries
- 4 tablespoons cocoa or cacao powder Cacao nibs Granola Hemp hearts To serve: Optional

Directions:

Combine all ingredients into a blender and blend until the desired smoothness is achieved. Pour into 2 tall glasses and serve topped with optional ingredients.

Cooked Iced Tea

Time To Prepare: two minutes
Time to Cook: 4 minutes
Yield: Servings 4

Ingredients:
- 2 tbsp. honey 4 regular tea bags 6 cups water

Directions:
1. Put in ingredients to the instant pot. Secure the lid.
2. Cook on HIGH pressure for 4 minutes. When done, depressurize naturally. Allow to cool to room temperature.
3. Serve over ice.

Cucumber Melon Smoothie

Time To Prepare: five minutes

Time to Cook: 0 minutes

Yield: Servings 2

Ingredients:
- 1 ½ cups of chopped honeydew
- 1 cup of chilled coconut water
- 1 cup of seedless cucumber, diced
- 2 tbsp. of fresh mint
- 6 to 8 ice cubes

Directions:

1. Mix the smoothie ingredients in your high-speed blender.

2. Pulse the ingredients a few times to cut them up.

3. Combine the mixture on the highest speed setting for thirty to 60 seconds.

4. Pour into glasses and serve.

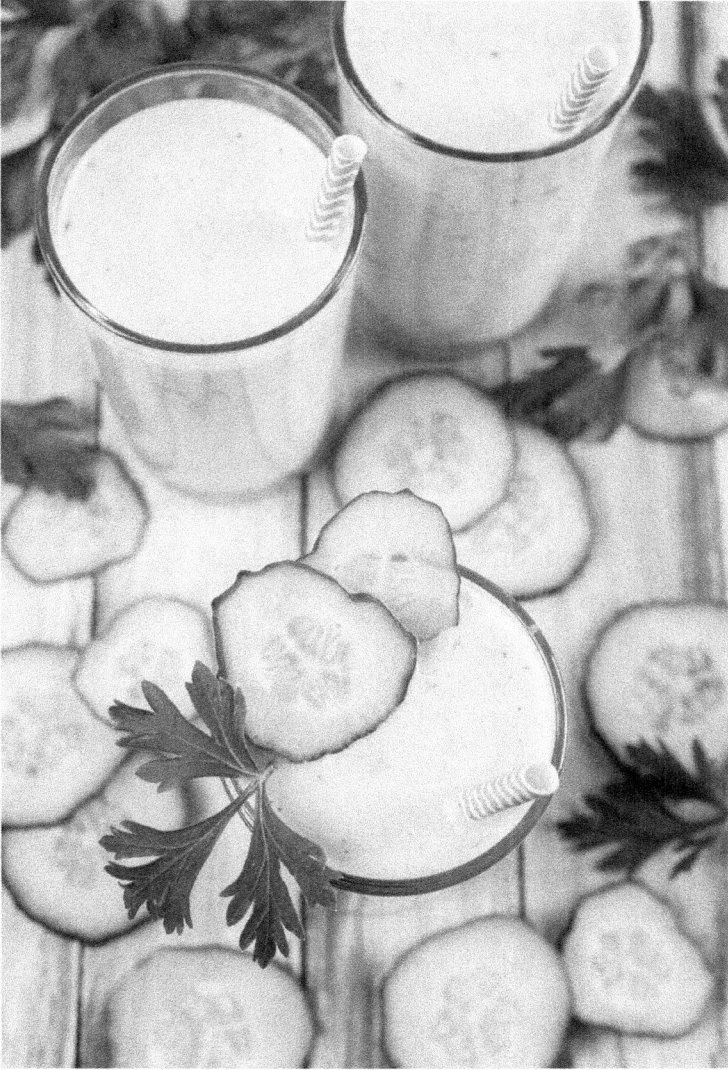

MEAT

Beef with Mushroom & Broccoli

Yield: 4 servings
Preparation Time: quarter-hour
Cooking Time: 12 minutes

Ingredients:
For Beef Marinade:
- 1 garlic clove, minced
- 1 (2-inch) piece fresh ginger, minced
- Salt and freshly ground black pepper, to taste
- 3 tablespoons white wine vinegar
- ¾ cup beef broth
- 1 pound flank steak, trimmed and sliced into thin strips

For Vegetables:
- 2 tablespoons coconut oil, divided
- 2 minced garlic cloves
- 3 cups broccoli rabe, chopped
- 4-ounce shiitake mushrooms, halved
- 8-ounce cremini mushrooms, sliced

Directions:
1. For marinade in a substantial bowl, mix together all ingredients except beef.

2. Add beef and coat with marinade generously.

3. Refrigerate to marinate for around quarter-hour.

4. In a substantial skillet, heat oil on medium-high heat.

5. Remove beef from bowl, reserving the marinade.

6. Add beef and garlic and cook for about 3-4 minutes or till browned.

7. With a slotted spoon, transfer the beef in a bowl.

8. In exactly the same skillet, add reserved marinade, broccoli and mushrooms and cook for approximately 3-4 minutes.

9. Stir in beef and cook for about 3-4 minutes.

Beef with Zucchini Noodles

Yield: 4 servings
Preparation Time: 15 minutes
Cooking Time: 9 minutes

Ingredients:
- 1 teaspoon fresh ginger, grated
- 2 medium garlic cloves, minced
- ¼ cup coconut aminos
- 2 tablespoons fresh lime juice
- 1½ pound NY strip steak, trimmed and sliced thinly
- 2 medium zucchinis, spiralized with Blade C
- Salt, to taste • 3 tablespoons essential olive oil
- 2 medium scallions, sliced
- 1 teaspoon red pepper flakes, crushed
- 2 tablespoons fresh cilantro, chopped

Directions:
1. In a big bowl, mix together ginger, garlic, coconut aminos and lime juice.
2. Add beef and coat with marinade generously.
3. Refrigerate to marinate approximately 10 minutes.
4. Place zucchini noodles over a large paper towel and sprinkle with salt.
5. Keep aside for around 10 minutes.
6. In a big skillet, heat oil on medium-high heat.
7. Add scallion and red pepper flakes and sauté for about 1 minute.

8. Add beef with marinade and stir fry for around 3-4 minutes or till browned.

9. Add zucchini and cook for approximately 3-4 minutes.

10. Serve hot with all the topping of cilantro.

Spiced Ground Beef

Yield: 5 servings
Preparation Time: 10 min
Cooking Time: 22 minutes

Ingredients:

- 2 tablespoons coconut oil
- 2 whole cloves
- 2 whole cardamoms
- 1 (2-inch) piece cinnamon stick
- 2 bay leaves
- 1 teaspoon cumin seeds
- 2 onions, chopped
- Salt, to taste
- ½ tablespoon garlic paste
- ½ tablespoon fresh ginger paste
- 1 pound lean ground beef
- 1½ teaspoons fennel seeds powder
- 1 teaspoon ground cumin
- 1½ teaspoons red chili powder
- 1/8 teaspoon ground turmeric
- Freshly ground black pepper, to taste
- 1 cup coconut milk

- ¼ cup water
- ¼ cup fresh cilantro, chopped

Directions:

1. In a sizable pan, heat oil on medium heat.
2. Add cloves, cardamoms, cinnamon stick, bay leaves and cumin seeds and sauté for about 20- a few seconds.
3. Add onion and 2 pinches of salt and sauté for about 3-4 minutes.
4. Add garlic-ginger paste and sauté for about 2 minutes.
5. Add beef and cook for about 4-5 minutes, entering pieces using the spoon.
6. Cover and cook for approximately 5 minutes.
7. Stir in spices and cook, stirring for approximately 2-2½ minutes.
8. Stir in coconut milk and water and cook for about 7-8 minutes.
9. Season with salt and take away from heat.
10. Serve hot using the garnishing of cilantro.

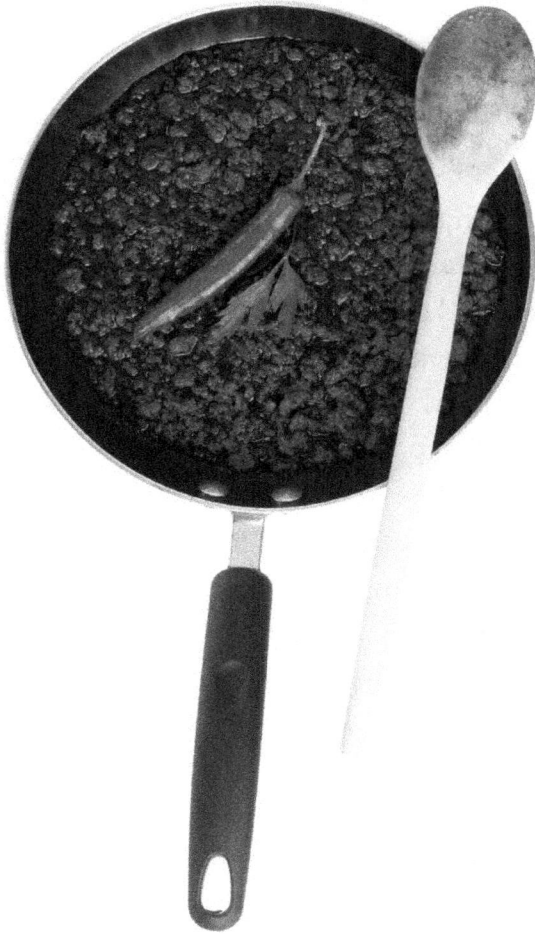

Ground Beef with Veggies

Yield: 2-4 servings

Preparation Time: quarter-hour

Cooking Time: twenty or so minutes

Ingredients

- 1-2 tablespoons coconut oil
- 1 red onion, sliced
- 2 red jalapeño peppers, seeded and sliced
- 2 minced garlic cloves
- 1 pound lean ground beef
- 1 small head broccoli, chopped
- ½ of head cauliflower, chopped
- 3 carrots, peeled and sliced
- 3 celery ribs, sliced
- Chopped fresh thyme, to taste
- Dried sage, to taste
- Ground turmeric, to taste
- Salt and freshly ground black pepper, to taste

Directions:

1. In a large skillet, melt coconut oil on medium heat.

2. Add onion, jalapeño peppers and garlic and sauté for about 5 minutes.

3. Add beef and cook for around 4-5 minutes, entering pieces using the spoon.

4. Add remaining ingredients and cook, stirring occasionally for about 8-10 min.

5. Serve hot.

Ground Beef with Greens & Tomatoes

Yield: 4 servings

Preparation Time: fifteen minutes

Cooking Time: 15 minutes

Ingredients:
- 1 tbsp organic olive oil
- ½ of white onion, chopped
- 2 garlic cloves, chopped finely
- 1 jalapeño pepper, chopped finely
- 1 pound lean ground beef
- 1 teaspoon ground coriander
- 1 teaspoon ground cumin
- ½ teaspoon ground turmeric
- ½ teaspoon ground ginger
- ½ teaspoon ground cinnamon
- ½ teaspoon ground fennel seeds
- Salt and freshly ground black pepper, to taste
- 8 fresh cherry tomatoes, quartered
- 8 collard greens leaves, stemmed and chopped
- 1 teaspoon fresh lemon juice

Directions:
1. In a big skillet, heat oil on medium heat.
2. Add onion and sauté for approximately 4 minutes.

3. Add garlic and jalapeño pepper and sauté for approximately 1 minute.

4. Add beef and spices and cook for approximately 6 minutes, breaking into pieces while using spoon.

5. Stir in tomatoes and greens and cook, stirring gently for about 4 minutes.

6. Stir in lemon juice and take away from heat.

Ground Beef & Veggies Curry

Yield: 6-8 servings

Preparation Time: 15 minutes

Cooking Time: 36 minutes

Ingredients:
- 2-3 tablespoons coconut oil
- 1 cup onion, chopped
- 1 garlic cloves, minced
- 1 pound lean ground beef
- 1½ tablespoons curry powder
- 1/8 teaspoon ground ginger
- 1/8 teaspoon ground cinnamon
- 1/8 teaspoon ground turmeric
- Salt, to taste
- 2½-3 cups tomatoes, chopped finely
- 2½-3 cups fresh peas, shelled
- 2 sweet potatoes, peeled and chopped

Directions:

1. In a sizable pan, melt coconut oil on medium heat.

2. Add onion and garlic and sauté for around 4-5 minutes.

3. Add beef and cook for about 4-5 minutes.

4. Add curry powder and spices and cook for about 1 minute.

5. Stir in tomatoes, peas and sweet potato and bring to your gentle simmer.

6. Simmer, covered approximately 25 minutes.

Curried Beef Meatballs

Yield: 6 servings
Preparation Time: twenty minutes
Cooking Time: 22 minutes

Ingredients:
For Meatballs:
- 1 pound lean ground beef
- 2 organic eggs, bea1o
- 3 tablespoons red onion, minced
- ¼ cup fresh basil leaves, chopped
- 1 (1-inch) fresh ginger piece, chopped finely
- 4 garlic cloves, chopped finely
- 3 Thai bird's eye chilies, minced
- 1 teaspoon coconut sugar
- 1 tablespoon red curry paste
- Salt, to taste • 1 tablespoon fish sauce
- 2 tablespoons coconut oil

For Curry:
- 1 red onion, chopped
- Salt, to taste
- 4 garlic cloves, minced
- 1 (1- inch) fresh ginger piece, minced
- 2 Thai bird's eye chilies, minced
- tablespoons red curry paste
- 1 (14-ounce) coconut milk
- Salt and freshly ground black pepper, to taste

- Lime wedges, for serving

Directions:
1. For meatballs in a large bowl, add all ingredients except oil and mix till well combined.
2. Make small balls from mixture.
3. In a large skillet, melt coconut oil on medium heat.
4. Add meatballs and cook for about 3-5 minutes or till golden brown all sides.
5. Transfer the meatballs right into a bowl.
6. In the same skillet, add onion as well as a pinch of salt and sauté for around 5 minutes.
7. Add garlic, ginger and chilies and sauté for about 1 minute.
8. Add curry paste and sauté for around 1 minute.
9. Add coconut milk and meatballs and convey to some gentle simmer.
10. Reduce the warmth to low and simmer, covered for around 10 minutes.
11. Serve using the topping of lime wedges.

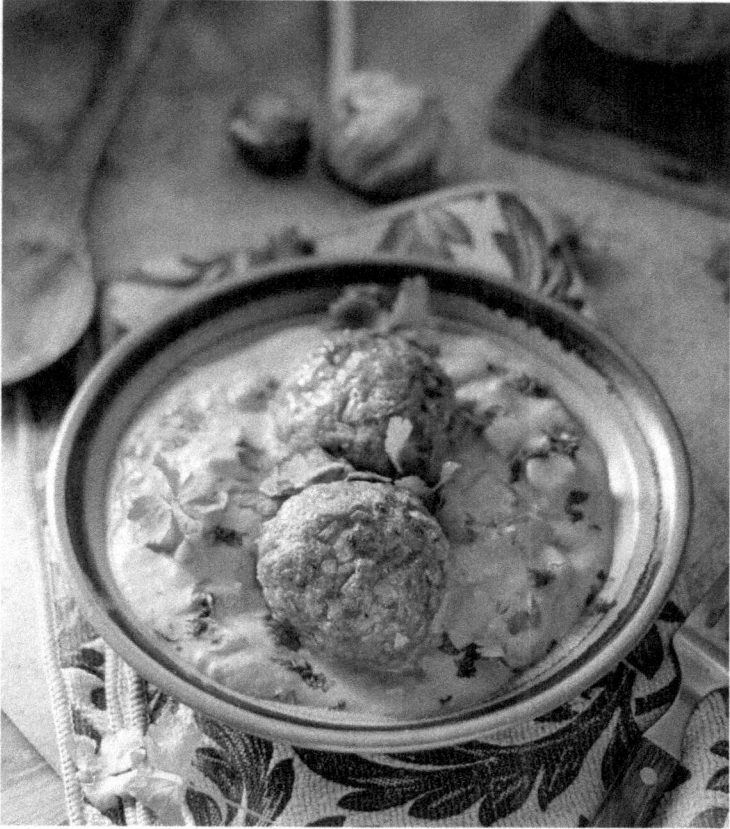

Honey Glazed Beef

Yield: 2-3 servings

Preparation Time: quarter-hour

Cooking Time: 12 minutes

Ingredients:
- 2 tablespoons arrowroot flour
- Salt and freshly ground black pepper, to taste
- 1 pound flank steak, cut into ¼-inch thick slices
- ½ cup plus 1 tablespoon coconut oil, divided
- 2 minced garlic cloves
- 1 teaspoon ground ginger
- Pinch of red pepper flakes, crushed
- 1/3 cup organic honey
- ½ cup beef broth
- ½ cup coconut aminos
- 3 scallions, chopped

Directions:

1. In a bowl, mix together arrowroot flour, salt and black pepper.

2. Coat beef slices in arrowroot flour mixture evenly after which get rid of excess mixture.Keep aside for about 10-15 minutes.

3. For sauce in a pan, melt 1 tablespoon of coconut oil on medium heat.

4. Add garlic, ginger powder and red pepper flakes and sauté for about 1 minute.

5. Add honey, broth and coconut aminos and stir to mix well.

6. Increase the heat to high and cook, stirring continuously for around 3 minutes. Remove from heat and keep aside.

7. In a large skillet, melt remaining coconut oil on medium heat.

8. Add beef and stir fry approximately 2-3 minutes.

9. Transfer the beef onto a paper towel lined plate to drain.

10. Remove the oil from skillet and return the beef into skillet. Stir fry for around 1 minute.

11. Stir in honey sauce and cook for approximately 3 minutes.

12. Stir in scallion and cook approximately 1 minute more.

13. Serve hot.

Grilled Skirt Steak Coconut

Yield: 4 servings

Preparation Time: quarter-hour

Cooking Time: 8-9 minutes

Ingredients:
- 2 teaspoons fresh ginger herb, grated finely
- 2 teaspoons fresh lime zest, grated finely
- ¼ cup coconut sugar
- 2 teaspoons fish sauce
- 2 tablespoons fresh lime juice
- ½ cup coconut milk
- 1 pound beef skirt steak, trimmed and cut into 4- inch slices lengthwise
- Salt, to taste

Directions:

1. In a sizable sealable bag, mix together all ingredients except steak and salt.

2. Add steak and coat with marinade generously.

3. Seal the bag and refrigerate to marinate for about 4-12 hours.

4. Preheat the grill to high heat. Grease the grill grate.

5. Remove steak from refrigerator and discard the marinade.

6. With a paper towel, dry the steak and sprinkle with salt evenly.

7. Cook the steak for approximately 3½ minutes.

8. Flip the medial side and cook for around 2½-5 minutes or till desired doneness.

9. Remove from grill pan and keep aside for approximately 5 minutes before slicing.

With a clear, crisp knife cut into desired slices and serve.

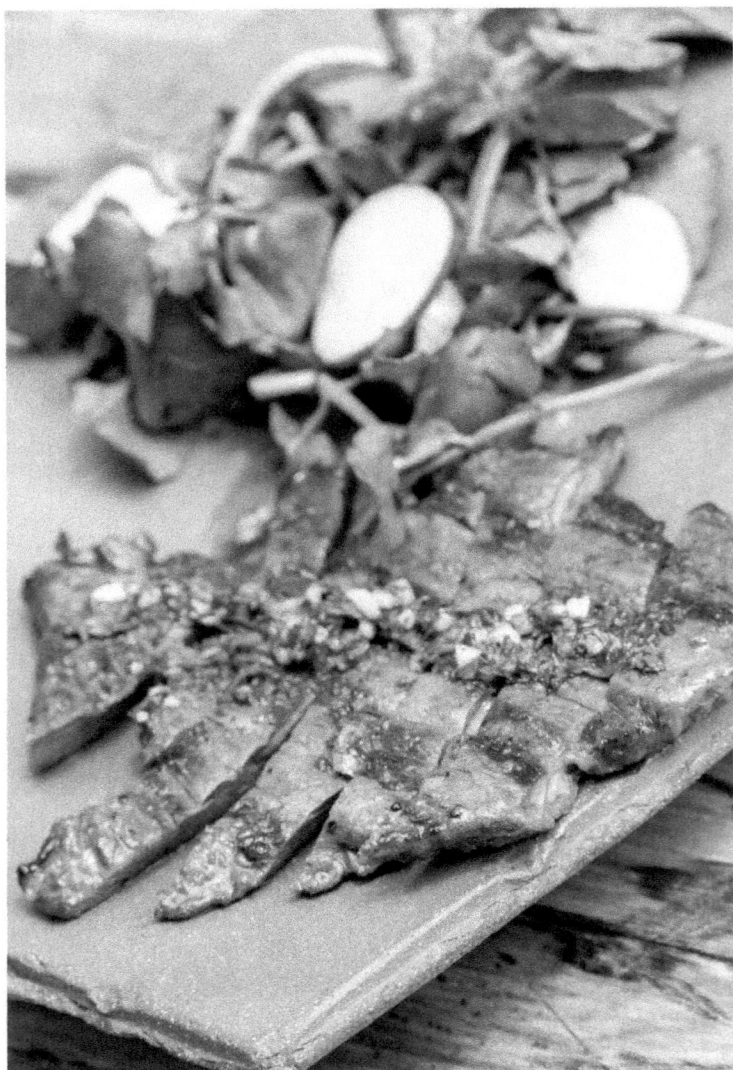

Lamb with Prunes

Yield: 4-6 servings

Preparation Time: fifteen minutes

Cooking Time: a couple of hours 40 minutes

Directions:

- 3 tablespoons coconut oil
- 2 onions, chopped finely
- 1 (1-inch) piece fresh ginger, minced
- 3 garlic cloves, minced
- ½ teaspoon ground turmeric
- 2 ½ pound lamb shoulder, trimmed and cubed into 3-inch size
- Salt and freshly ground black pepper, to taste
- ½ teaspoon saffron threads, crumbled
- 1 cinnamon stick
- 3 cups water
- 1 cup runes, pitted and halved

Directions:

1. In a big pan, melt coconut oil on medium heat.

2. Add onions, ginger, garlic cloves and turmeric and sauté for about 3-5 minutes.

3. Sprinkle the lamb with salt and black pepper evenly.

4. In the pan, add lamb and saffron threads and cook for approximately 4-5 minutes.

5. Add cinnamon stick and water and produce to some boil on high heat.

6. Reduce the temperature to low and simmer, covered for around 1½-120 minutes or till desired doneness of lamb.
7. Stir in prunes and simmer for approximately 20-a half-hour.
8. Remove cinnamon stick and serve hot.

Baked Lamb with Spinach

Yield: 6 servings
Preparation Time: quarter-hour
Cooking Time: couple of hours 55 minutes

Ingredients:
- 2 tablespoons coconut oil
- 2 pound lamb necks, trimmed and cut into 2-inch pieces crosswise
- Salt, to taste
- 2 medium onions, chopped
- 3 tablespoons fresh ginger, minced
- 4 garlic cloves, minced
- 2 tablespoons ground coriander
- 1 tablespoon ground cumin
- 1 teaspoon ground turmeric
- ¼ cup coconut milk
- ½ cup tomatoes, chopped
- 2 cups boiling water
- 30-ounce frozen spinach, thawed and squeezed
- 1½ tablespoons garam masala
- 1 tablespoon fresh lemon juice
- Freshly ground black pepper, to taste

Directions:

1. Preheat the oven to 300 degrees F.

2. In a substantial Dutch oven, melt coconut oil on medium-high heat.

3. Add lamb necks and sprinkle with salt.

4. Stir fry approximately 4-5 minutes or till browned completely.

5. Transfer the lamb right into a plate and lower the heat to medium.

6. In exactly the same pan, add onion and sauté for about 10 minutes.

7. Add ginger, garlic and spices and sauté for around 1 minute.

8. Add coconut milk and tomatoes and cook approximately 3-4 minutes.

9. With an immersion blender, blend the mix till smooth.

10. Add lamb, boiling water and salt and convey to some boil.

11. Cover the pan and transfer into the oven. Bake for approximately 2½ hours.

12. Now, take away the pan from oven and place on medium heat.

13. Stir in spinach and garam masala and cook for about 3-5 minutes.

14. Stir in fresh lemon juice, salt and black pepper and take off from heat.

15. Serve hot.

DESSERTS

Pumpkin Ice Cream

Time To Prepare: fifteen minutes
Time to Cook: 0 minutes
Yield: Servings 6

Ingredients:
- ½ cup of dates (pitted and chopped)
- ½ teaspoon of ground cinnamon
- ½ teaspoon of vanilla flavor
- 1 (fifteen-ounce) can of sugar-free pumpkin puree
- 1 ½ teaspoon of pumpkin pie spice
- 2 (14-ounce) cans of unsweetened coconut milk
- Pinch of salt

Directions:
1. Combine all ingredients in a high-speed blender and pulse.
2. Move the puree to an airtight container and freeze for roughly 1-2 hours.
3. Move the frozen puree to an ice-cream maker and process following the manufacturers.
4. Return the ice cream to the airtight container and freeze for approximately 1-2 hours before you serve.

Raspberry Diluted Frozen Sorbet

Time To Prepare: 10 min
Time to Cook: 20 min
Yield: Servings 4

Ingredients:
- 1 tsp honey 14oz / 400g frozen raspberry fl oz / 50g almond milk Mint

Directions:
1. Place the almond milk and raspberry in a mixer till it's smooth and leave the consistency in the freezer for about twenty minutes.
2. When serving, place them in ice cream bowls and serve with mint on top.

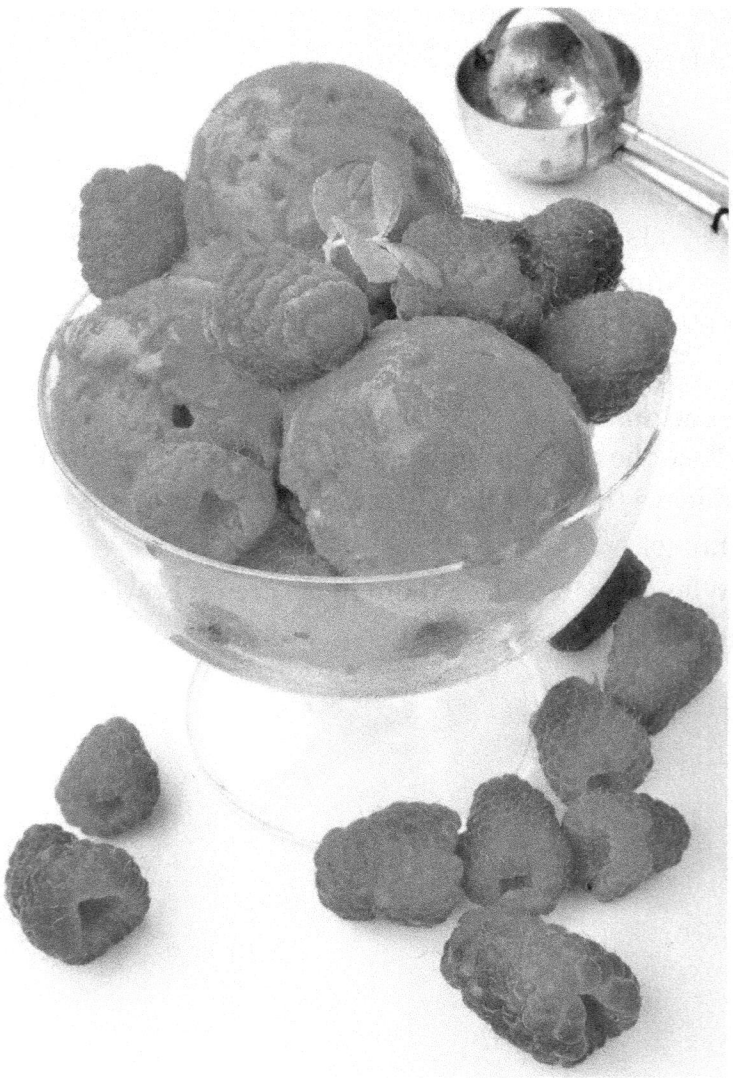

Raspberry Gummies

Time To Prepare:five minutes
Time to Cook: fifteen minutes
Yield: Servings 6

Ingredients:
- ¼ cup of grass-fed gelatin
- ¾ cup of cold water
- 1 cup of frozen raspberries
- 3 tablespoons of raw honey

Directions:
1. Pour water into a blender followed by frozen raspberries.
2. Puree and move them to a deep cooking pan on moderate heat.
3. Put in honey and gelatin. Whisk. Reduce the heat, then whisk constantly for five minutes.
4. Place the mixture on a baking dish or molds and place in your fridge for 60 minutes or until it firms. If you used a baking dish, chop the gelatin into squares. Pop the gelatin out with the molds.

Refreshing Raspberry Jelly

Time To Prepare: ten minutes+ 1 hour freezing
Time to Cook: thirty minutes
Yield: Servings 4

Ingredients:
- ¼ cup of water
- 1 tbsp. of fresh lemon juice
- 2 pound of fresh raspberries

Directions:
1. In a moderate-sized pan, put in raspberries and water on low heat and cook for approximately 8-ten minutes until done completely.
2. Put in lemon juice and cook for approximately 30 minutes, stirring once in a while. Turn off the heat and put the mixture into a sieve.
3. Position a strainer over a container. Through strainer, strain the mixture by pushing using the backside of a spoon.
4. Place the mixture into a blender then pulse till a jelly-like texture is formed.
5. Move into serving glass bowls and place in your fridge for minimum for approximately 1 hour.

Rum Butter Cookies

Time To Prepare: ten minutes + chilling time
Time to Cook: five minutes
Yield: Servings 12

Ingredients:
- ½ cup coconut butter
- ½ cup confectioners' Swerve
- 1 stick butter
- 1 teaspoon rum extract 4 cups almond meal

Directions:
1. Melt the coconut butter and butter.
2. Mix in the Swerve and rum extract.
3. Afterward, put in the almond meal and mix to blend.
4. Roll the balls and put them on a parchment-lined cookie sheet.
5. Keep in your fridge until ready to serve.

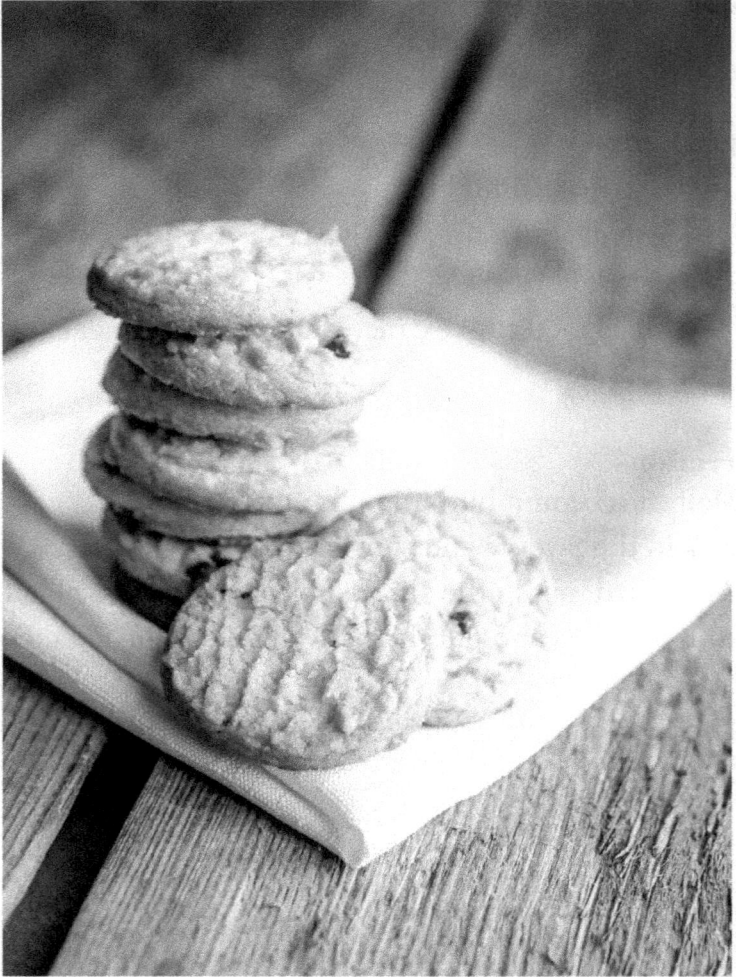

Spiced Tea Pudding

Time To Prepare: ten minutes
Time to Cook: ten minutes
Yield: Servings 3

Ingredients:
- ½ cup coconut flakes
- ½ teaspoon cloves
- 1 ½ cups berries
- 1 can coconut milk
- 1 cup almond milk
- 1 tablespoon chia seeds
- 1 tablespoon ground cinnamon
- 1 tablespoon raw honey
- 1 teaspoon allspice
- 1 teaspoon cardamom
- 1 teaspoon green tea powder
- 1 teaspoon nutmeg
- 2 tablespoons pumpkin seeds
- 2 teaspoons ground ginger

Directions:
1. In your blender, puree tea powder with coconut milk, almond milk, cinnamon, coconut flakes, nutmeg, allspice, cloves, honey, cardamom, and ginger split into bowls.
2. Heat a pan on moderate heat, put in berries until bubbling, then move to your blender and pulse well.

3. Split the berries into the bowls with the coconut milk mix, top with chia seeds and pumpkin seeds before you serve. Enjoy!

Strawberry Granita

Time To Prepare: ten minutes
Time to Cook: ten minutes
Yield: Servings 8

Ingredients:
- ¼ teaspoon balsamic vinegar
- ½ teaspoon lemon juice
- 1 cup of water
- 2 lb. strawberries, halved & hulled Agave to taste
- Just a small pinch of salt

Directions:
1. Wash the strawberries in water. Keep in a blender. Put in water, agave, balsamic vinegar, salt, and lemon juice. Pulse multiple times so that the mixture moves. Blend until smooth.
2. Pour into a baking dish. The puree must be 3/8 inch deep only.
3. Place in your fridge the dish uncovered till the edges start to freeze. The center must be slushy. Stir crystals from the edges lightly into the center. Stir thoroughly to mix. Chill till the granite is nearly fully frozen. Scrape loose the crystals like before and mix. Place in your fridge once more. Using a fork, stir 3-4 times till the granite has become light.

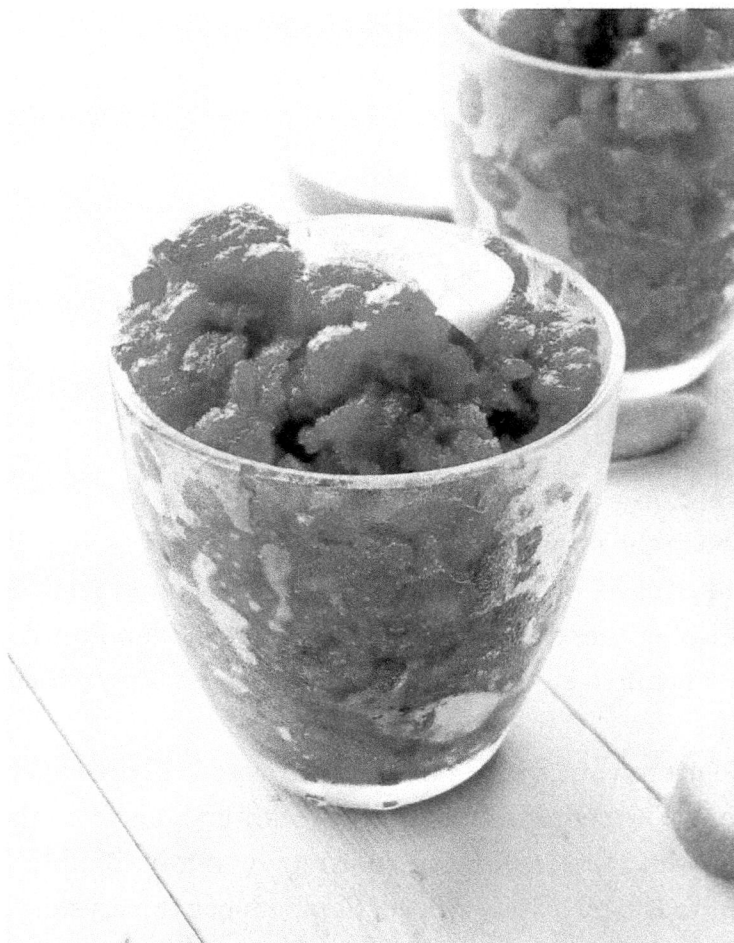

Strawberry Orange Sorbet

Time To Prepare: five minutes
Time to Cook: 0 minutes
Yield: Servings 3

Ingredients:

- 1 cup Orange juice or coconut water
- 1 pound Frozen strawberries

Direction:

1. Pour strawberries in a blender and pulse until all you have left are flakes. two minutes tops.

2. Now put in the coconut water or orange juice and pulse until you get a nice and smooth puree. Have a spatula handy because you might need to scrape some of the puree off the walls of the blender sometimes.

3. Serve the moment you're done or put in the freezer for about forty-five minutes for a sorbet feel.

4. Also, you can pour the smoothie into popsicle molds and freeze for hours or even overnight. Enjoy!

Strawberry Soufflé

Time To Prepare: fifteen minutes
Time to Cook: twelve minutes
Yield: Servings 6

Ingredients:
- 18 ounces of fresh strawberries hulled
- 5 organic egg whites, divided
- 4 teaspoons of fresh lemon juice
- 1/3 cup of raw honey, divided

Directions:
1. Preheat your oven to 350F.
2. Place the strawberries in a blender then pulse until a puree form.
3. Strain the strawberry puree using a strainer while discarding the seeds.
4. Mix the strawberry puree to three tablespoons of honey, two egg whites, and fresh lemon juice. Pulse until a frothy and light-weight develops.
5. Beat the eggs in a separate container until it becomes frothy. Put in the remaining honey and beat until a stiff peak forms.
6. Gently- fold the egg whites into the strawberry mixture.
7. Move the mixture to six big ramekins and place them on a baking sheet.
8. Bake for around 10-twelve minutes. Take out of the oven and serve instantly.

The Most Elegant Parsley Soufflé Ever

Time To Prepare: five minutes
Time to Cook: six minutes
Yield: Servings 5

Ingredients:
- 1 fresh red chili pepper, chopped
- 1 tablespoon fresh parsley, chopped
- 2 tablespoons coconut cream
- 2 whole eggs Sunflower seeds to taste

Directions:
1. Preheat the oven to 390 degrees F Almond butter 2 soufflé dishes
2. Place the ingredients to a blender and mix thoroughly
3 Split batter into soufflé dishes and bake for about six minutes
Serve and enjoy!

Tropical Popsicles

Time To Prepare: 10 Minutes
Time to Cook: 10 Minutes
Yield: Servings 6

Ingredients:
- ½ tsp. Black Pepper
- 2 Kiwi, cut
- 2 tbsp. Coconut Oil
- 2 tsp. Turmeric
- 3 cups Pineapple, chopped

Directions:
1. First, place all the ingredients needed to make the popsicles excluding the kiwi in a high-speed blender for a couple of minutes or until you get a smooth mixture.
2. After this, pour the smoothie into the popsicle molds.
3. Next, insert the kiwi slices into the molds and then put the frames in the freezer until set.
Tip: If you desire texture, you can blend it less

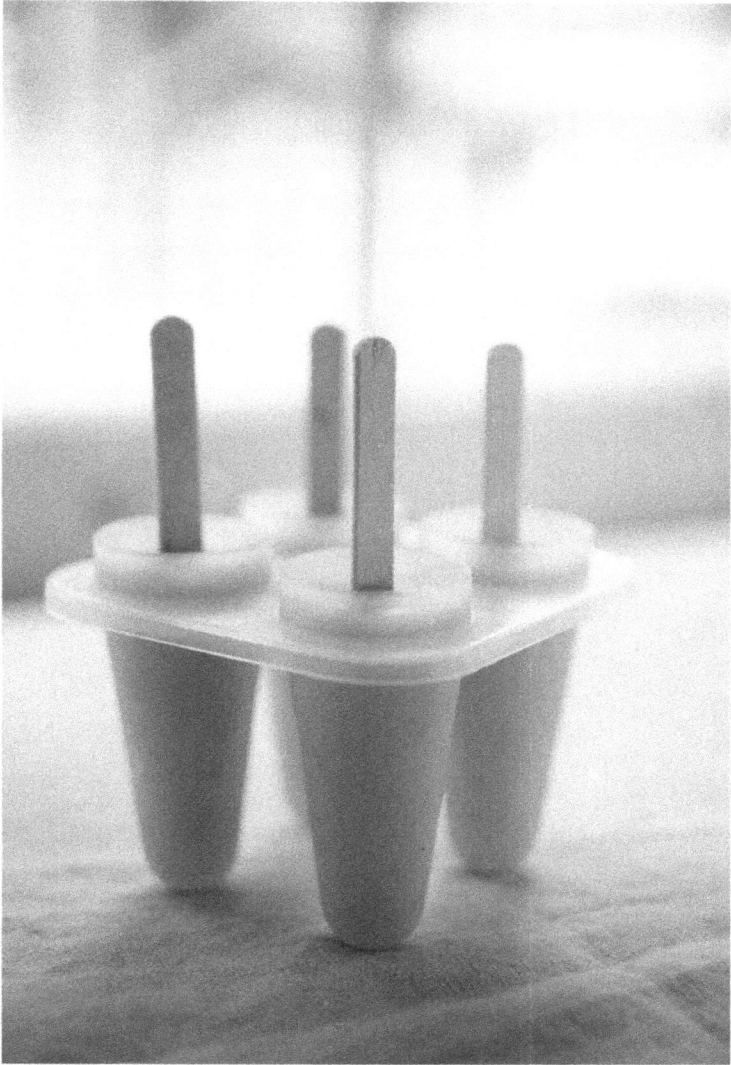